The Pan Asian Modified Mediterranean Diet Cookbook

Easy and Healthy PAMM Diet Recipes to Lose Weight and Prevent Diseases

Janda Blardon

Table of contents

Introduction

Let's reboot your lifestyle and cherish the great wealth of health by eating a balanced and healthy diet. A balanced diet is best defined by the range of nutrients it provides. There are many options on the cards, but the Pan-Asian Modified Mediterranean – PAMM diet guarantees a much-needed balance to the diet with a variety of its healthy and nutritious ingredients. This diet comes with a unique nutritional formula of its own, and this cookbook will let you unlock all of its secrets. Now you can cook delicious PAMM meals at home using a variety of recipes given here. Let us first take a look at how this diet actually works and what are factors make it extremely successful in achieving better health goals.

Chapter 1: What is Pan Asian Modified Mediterranean Diet?

The word PAMM was first coined by Dr. Stephen Sinatra, who also proposed the idea of modifying the original Mediterranean diet and fuse it with Chinese, Thai, and Japanese cuisines, and hence the word "Pan Asian" became the part of this term. The idea was to make this diet healthier than ever and bring more diversity in its flavors. Later, when the diet was practically used and implemented, it showed great health benefits. It is now coined as the best anti-inflammatory diet or sometimes called a heart-healthy diet. Due to the variety of flavors and meals the diet offers, it quickly received a welcoming response from people around the world.

The reason the PAMM diet has been able to ensure numerous health advantages is that it is designed with a nutritional formula. This formula sets a limit to the consumption of all the macronutrients, i.e., proteins, fats, and carbohydrates. The daily use of these macros is set according to the average body needs of a healthy human adult; thus, it can keep you healthy and active while preventing several health problems. Dr. Stephen not only proposed the idea of limited macros intake but also presented a list of PAMM food items that must be preferred for each meal.

- The Best Diet that Treats Inflammation

The PAMM diet works like a miracle when it comes to treating inflammation in the body. There are various causes of inflammation, from our lifestyle to our eating habits, and certain health conditions, anything can affect the body's responses which may lead to inflammation. Our diet is another factor that may aggravate the inflammatory condition due to the metabolic waste they produce after complete digestion or due to the agents that can trigger the body's inflammatory response. Thankfully, all the ingredients and food items that are prescribed in the PAMM diet have anti-inflammatory properties that may include fresh organic vegetables, spices, herbs, fresh fruits and it also discourages those food items which can cause inflammation in the body like processed meat, high carb meals, sugary snacks and good, etc.

- Other Health Benefits of PAMM Diet

PAMM diet is not only anti-inflammatory

o Lowering of Cholesterol

The PAMM diet suggests controlled fat intake, and these fats must be sourced from healthy sources. Healthy fats are categorized as monounsaturated or polyunsaturated fats, which are free from Low-density lipoproteins-LDL or bad cholesterol.

o Controlled Blood Pressure

High blood pressure results from a number of health problems, and an unhealthy high cholesterol diet is one factor that most contributes to high blood pressure as the bad cholesterols accumulate in the blood vessels and cause an obstruction in the flow of blood. PAMM diet due to its healthy and controlled fat intake keeps the blood pressure under control.

o Heart Healthy Diet

PAMM diet is highly beneficial for the people who are suffering from heart problems or have a tendency to have heart disease. This diet is capable of controlling cholesterol levels and blood pressure, which indirectly keeps the heart healthy and cardiac muscles strong.

o Increased Cellular Activity

PAMM diet provides all the much need elements which our cells require for their endless activities. Protein formation, replication, healing, and repair all the process which require a controlled and a constant supply of basic nutrients and energy. PAMM diet regulates the supply and provides energy through a well-regulated mechanism. It syncs well with cellular activities and increases their rate. Moreover, the diet helps in maintaining a conducive environment for accelerated cellular activity.

o Accelerated Metabolism

A diet rich in proteins, fats, carbs, fibers, vitamins, and minerals can quickly boost the rate of metabolism in the body. Our cells require an optimum supply of energy as well as proteins to carry out their cellular activities, and the PAMM diet ensures a constant and balanced supply of these nutrients. It can also regulate the production of enzymes and hormones in the body, which help accelerate the metabolic rates.

How Does the PAMM Diet Work?

The PAMM diet is not that restrictive as many other health-oriented diets are. It only emphasizes the right intake of the healthy ingredients in the right amount. The diet works through the balance it brings to the diet. According to Dr. Stephen's idea of the PAMM diet, it must contain:

- 20 to 25 percent lean protein
- 35 to 40 percent healthy fats
- 40 to 45 percent low-glycemic carbohydrates

And this basic limit set a series of obvious guidelines to follow. In order to maintain this proportion of the macronutrients, the dieter is forced to consume only rich and healthy ingredients. All the health-damaging ingredients are omitted out of the diet.

- Low Glycemic Carbohydrates

The instant source of energy, the carbohydrates, should only constitute 40 percent of this diet, which means that you can easily consume more of the carb-rich ingredients, but the only restriction is to opt low glycemic food only. The glycemic index of a food indicates the number of refined carbohydrates present in the food. The highest glycemic index is that of sugar, which is purely made out of refined carbohydrates. All other food items are then compared to it to calculate their relative glycemic values. On a scale of 0-100, the food items having glycemic index lower 50 are considered as low glycemic food. And according to the PAMM diet, the dieter can freely consume these low glycemic food items. Food with a higher glycemic index is not only unhealthy, but it also increases the overall percentage of carb intake in the meals; hence they must be avoided. The reason why refined carbohydrates are restricting on this diet is that they can instantly raise the blood sugar levels, which can lead to insulin resistance, diabetes, heart problems, and obesity in the longer run.

- Lean Proteins

Protein contains amino acids that are needed by every human cell to build and repair itself. Out of the 22 amino acids, the eight of them are essential, and they must be sourced from the food that we eat. And in order to meet this need, we must consider all the available options for protein intake. The best-known source of proteins is animal meat or other animal-based products. But not all forms of animal food are healthy, so some plant-based sources must also be used to increase the protein intake. PAMM encourages the use of whole grains, dairy products, white meat to regulate the protein intake, but red meat can only be consumed in a small amount since it is not healthy and contain saturated fats and toxins.

- Healthy Fats

The need for consuming healthy fats cannot be overemphasized. Fats play an important role in the body, from making membrane structures to the important organelles in the body. So, avoid fats altogether is not an option; however, we can regulate our health through the consumption of healthy fats. Like carbohydrates, fats also provide energy, but they are metabolized differently. By consuming fats that contain good cholesterol-high density lipoproteins, we can ensure good health. If you consume fats in a high amount, more than the body's energy requirement than the excess is accumulated in the blood vessels and other parts of the body, causing cardiac problems. But by controlling the intake to a 35 percent limit and restricting yourself only to healthy fats, all the risks of such diseases can be minimized and even prevented if the diet is followed on a long-term basis.

List of PAMM Food

Since the PAMM diet takes its roots from the Mediterranean diet, its list of food also reminds you of the healthy Mediterranean diet ingredients. The plus point is that it adds up a few more healthy options to the diet making it more diverse and richer. In this section, we will discover which category of food is best suited for the Pan Asian Modified Mediterranean Diet.

1. Vegetables

Vegetable which is rich in fibers and minerals are most suitable for this diet like broccoli, tomatoes, kale, onions, spinach, cauliflower, Brussels sprouts, cucumbers, etc. The starchy vegetables with a high glycemic load like potatoes, beets, and yams, etc. must be avoided, or their intake must be minimized to keep the carb intake balanced.

2. Fruits

Fruits with a glycemic index lower than 55 are considered appropriate for the PAMM diet that may include: pears, apples, oranges, strawberries, bananas, grapefruit, blueberries, blackberries, peaches, and prunes, etc.

3. Nuts and seeds

Nuts and seeds provide essential oils, vitamins, and minerals without adding many refined carbs to the diet; their intake is highly recommended on this diet. Nuts and seeds to add to your daily meal may include walnuts, almonds, hazelnuts, cashews, sunflower seeds, macadamia nuts, pumpkin seeds, etc.

4. Whole grains

Focus more on whole grains and increase their consumption as they contain a perfect balance of complex carbs, proteins, and fibers. Widely recommended whole grains include oats, brown rice, rye, buckwheat, barley, corn, whole-grain bread, whole wheat, and pasta.

5. Fish and seafood

Seafood is always considered a safe choice as it is rich in proteins and omega 3 and 6. The seafood that we can freely add to our PAMM diet includes sardines, salmon, tuna, trout, mussels, mackerel, oysters, clams, shrimp, crab, etc. Fresh seafood is preferable over processed or canned ones.

6. Poultry

White meat is broadly considered healthy; it is rich in proteins and does not contain any toxins. Chicken, turkey, duck, etc. are some of the options that you can try on this diet.

7. Eggs

Eggs are known as a complete diet of their own and do not only contain proteins but a number of other minerals and vitamins too. Having eggs on this diet is the easiest and quickest means of meeting all your protein needs.

8. Dairy

Dairy products that can provide minimum carbs are considered healthier for consumption on the PAMM diet. The dieter can freely consume a variety of cheese, yogurt, yogurt, cream cheese, and cream, etc. Remember to consume these ingredients while keeping the nutritional intake in a balance.

9. Herbs and spices

There is no harm in consuming a variety of herbs and spices; rather, it is considered healthy as spices can trigger more enzyme production. On this diet, you have garlic powder, basil, mint, rosemary, sage, nutmeg, cinnamon, pepper, and all other powdered and whole spices and herbs, etc.

10. Healthy Fats

Fats that have low cholesterol and contain unsaturated fatty acids are termed as healthy and for PAMM diet following fats options are suitable for daily intake: extra virgin olive oil, and avocado oil.

Chapter 2: Meal Plan

Day 1

Breakfast: Pineapple & Mango Smoothie

Lunch: Meatballs & Quinoa Bowl

Dinner: Tuna with Olives

Day 2

Breakfast: Blueberry & Ricotta Toast

Lunch: Veggie Tortillas

Dinner: Roasted Chicken

Day 3

Breakfast: Quinoa Porridge

Lunch: Watermelon & Cucumber Salad

Dinner: Salmon with Avocado Cream

Day 4

Breakfast: Banana & Blueberry Muffins

Lunch: Pasta with Tomatoes

Dinner: Salmon & Beans Salad

Day 5

Breakfast: Kale & Tomato Scramble

Lunch: Pita Sandwiches

Dinner: Braised Chicken

Day 6

Breakfast: Oatmeal Pancakes

Lunch: Pasta with Tomatoes

Dinner: Chicken & Veggie Salad

Day 7

Breakfast: Berries & Beet Smoothie Bowl

Lunch: Chickpeas Wraps

Dinner: Braised Chicken

Day 8

Breakfast: Overnight Oatmeal

Lunch: Berries & Mango Salad

Dinner: Chicken & Chickpeas Stew

Day 9

Breakfast: Eggs with Spinach

Lunch: Nutty Quinoa

Dinner: Salmon with Avocado Cream

Day 10

Breakfast: Oatmeal & Yogurt Bowl

Lunch: Turkey Burgers

Dinner: Lentil & Spinach Soup

Day 11

Breakfast: Banana & Blueberry Muffins

Lunch: Lentil Falafel Bowl

Dinner: Chicken with Spinach & Pasta

Day 12

Breakfast: Berries Yogurt Bowl

Lunch: Pasta & Tomato Salad

Dinner: Braised Chicken

Day 13

Breakfast: Eggs with Spinach

Lunch: Meatballs & Quinoa Bowl

Dinner: Lentil & Spinach Soup

Day 14

Breakfast: Cherry & Blueberry Smoothie

Lunch: Spaghetti with Broccoli

Dinner: Nutty Chicken Salad

Day 15

Breakfast: Oatmeal Pancakes

Lunch: Greens Salad

Dinner: Salmon with Capers Sauce

Day 16

Breakfast: Berry Yogurt Bowl

Lunch: Chicken & Veggie Skewers

Dinner: Lentil & Quinoa Casserole

Day 17

Breakfast: Kale & Tomato Scramble

Lunch: Pita Sandwiches

Dinner: Tuna Salad

Day 18

Breakfast: Quinoa Porridge

Lunch: Turkey Burgers

Dinner: Chickpeas & Veggie Curry

Day 19

Breakfast: Oatmeal & Yogurt Bowl

Lunch: Mango, Avocado & Greens Salad

Dinner: Roasted Chicken

Day 20

Breakfast: Blueberry & Ricotta Toast

Lunch: Lentil Falafel Bowl

Dinner: Salmon with Capers Sauce

Day 21

Breakfast: Berries & Spinach Smoothie

Lunch: Chicken & Veggie Skewers

Dinner: Lentil & Quinoa Casserole

Chapter 3: Smoothies Recipes

Berries & Spinach Smoothie

Preparation Time: 10 minutes
Servings: 2

Ingredients:

- 1½ cups mixed frozen berries (blueberries, strawberries, cranberries)
- 2 cups fresh spinach
- 1 cup celery stalk, chopped
- 1 (2-inch) pieces fresh ginger, peeled and chopped
- 3 tablespoons hemp protein powder
- 1¼ cups filtered water

Method:

1. Add all ingredients in a high-power blender and pulse until smooth.
2. Pour into two glasses and serve immediately.

Nutritional Information per Serving:

- Calories 122
- Total Fat 1.7 g
- Saturated Fat 0.1 g
- Cholesterol 0 mg
- Sodium 64 mg
- Total Carbs 20.4 g
- Fiber 7.5 g
- Sugar 0.1 g
- Protein 6.4 g

Strawberry Oatmeal Smoothie

Preparation Time: 10 minutes

Servings: 2

Ingredients:

- ½ cup gluten-free rolled oats
- 2 cups frozen strawberries
- 1 banana, peeled and sliced
- 1 teaspoon chia seeds
- ½ teaspoon vanilla extract
- 6 ounces plain Greek yogurt
- ½ cup unsweetened almond milk

Method:

1. Add all ingredients in a high-power blender and pulse until smooth.
2. Pour the smoothie into two glasses and serve immediately.

Nutritional Information per Serving:

- Calories 293
- Total Fat 8.5 g
- Saturated Fat 3.6 g
- Cholesterol 19 mg
- Sodium 102 mg
- Total Carbs 49.2 g
- Fiber 7.7 g
- Sugar 21.9 g
- Protein 8 g

Strawberry & Beet Smoothie

Preparation Time: 10 minutes
Servings: 2

Ingredients:

- 2 cups frozen strawberries, pitted and chopped
- 2/3 cup roasted and frozen beet, chopped
- 1 teaspoon fresh ginger, peeled and grated
- 1 teaspoon fresh turmeric, peeled and grated
- ½ cup fresh orange juice
- 1 cup unsweetened almond milk

Method:

1. Add all ingredients in a high-power blender and pulse until smooth.
2. Pour the smoothie into two glasses and serve immediately.

Nutritional Information per Serving:

- Calories 126
- Total Fat 2.6 g
- Saturated Fat 0.2 g
- Cholesterol 0 mg
- Sodium 136 mg
- Total Carbs 25.5 g
- Fiber 5 g
- Sugar 16.8 g
- Protein 3 g

Cherry & Blueberry Smoothie

Preparation Time: 10 minutes

Servings: 2

Ingredients:

- ½ cup frozen blueberries
- ½ cup frozen cherries
- 2 cups fresh baby kale
- ¼ teaspoon ground cinnamon
- ¼ teaspoon ground turmeric
- 1 scoop chocolate protein powder
- 1 cup filtered water
- 5 ice cubes, crushed

Method:

1. Add all ingredients in a high-power blender and pulse until smooth.
2. Pour the smoothie into two glasses and serve immediately.

Nutritional Information per Serving:

- Calories 172
- Total Fat 1.1 g
- Saturated Fat 0.6 g
- Cholesterol 21 mg
- Sodium 116 mg
- Total Carbs 29.3 g
- Fiber 3.9 g
- Sugar 17.8 g
- Protein 13.8 g

Cherry & Spinach Smoothie

Preparation Time: 10 minutes
Servings: 2

Ingredients:

- 2 ripe bananas, peeled and sliced
- 1 cup fresh cherries, pitted
- 2 cups fresh spinach
- 1 teaspoon fresh ginger, peeled and chopped
- 1 tablespoon almonds
- ½ teaspoon ground turmeric
- ¼ teaspoon ground cinnamon
- 1½ cups chilled filtered water

Method:

1. Add all ingredients in a high-power blender and pulse until smooth.
2. Pour the smoothie into two glasses and serve immediately.

Nutritional Information per Serving:

- Calories 250
- Total Fat 2.3 g
- Saturated Fat 0.3 g
- Cholesterol 0 mg
- Sodium 27 mg
- Total Carbs 58.9 g
- Fiber 7.2 g
- Sugar 41 g
- Protein 4.4 g

Mango & Strawberry Smoothie

Preparation Time: 0 minutes

Servings: 2

Ingredients:

- 1 large frozen banana, peeled and sliced
- 1 cup frozen strawberries
- ½ cup frozen mango
- ¼ teaspoon ground turmeric
- ¼ teaspoon ground ginger
- 1 tablespoon honey
- ½ cup plain Greek yogurt
- ½ cup unsweetened almond milk

Method:

1. Add all ingredients in a high-power blender and pulse until smooth.
2. Pour into two glasses and serve immediately.

Nutritional Information per Serving:

- Calories 188
- Total Fat 2.2 g
- Saturated Fat 0.8 g
- Cholesterol 4 mg
- Sodium 90 mg
- Total Carbs 39 g
- Fiber 4 g
- Sugar 29.3 g
- Protein 5.3 g

Pineapple & Mango Smoothie

Preparation Time: 10 minutes
Servings: 2

Ingredients:

- 1½ cups mango, peeled, pitted and chopped
- 1½ cups pineapple, peeled and chopped
- 1 tablespoon chia seeds
- 1 teaspoon ground turmeric
- ½ teaspoon ground ginger
- ½ teaspoon ground cinnamon
- 1½ cups coconut milk
- ¼ cup ice cubes

Method:

1. Add all the ingredients in a high-power blender and pulse until creamy.
2. Pour the smoothie into two glasses and serve immediately.

Nutritional Information per Serving:

- Calories 457
- Total Fat 32 g
- Saturated Fat 27.3 g
- Cholesterol 0 mg
- Sodium 78 mg
- Total Carbs 46.8 g
- Fiber 5.6 g
- Sugar 32.2 g
- Protein 4.1 g

Mango & Spinach Smoothie

Preparation Time: 10 minutes
Servings: 2

Ingredients:

- 2 cups frozen mango, peeled, pitted and chopped
- 3 cups fresh spinach, chopped
- 1 teaspoon ground turmeric
- 1 teaspoon fresh lemon juice
- 1 teaspoon fresh lime juice
- 16 ounces fresh coconut water

Method:

1. Add all ingredients in a high-power blender and pulse until smooth.
2. Pour the smoothie into two glasses and serve immediately.

Nutritional Information per Serving:

- Calories 114
- Total Fat 0.9 g
- Saturated Fat 0.2 g
- Cholesterol 0 mg
- Sodium 318 mg
- Total Carbs 27.1 g
- Fiber 3.9 g
- Sugar 22.8 g
- Protein 2.8 g

Spinach & Cucumber Smoothie

Preparation Time: 10 minutes
Servings: 2

Ingredients:

- 1 large frozen banana, peeled and sliced
- 3 cups fresh spinach leaves
- 1 cucumber, peeled and chopped
- 2 tablespoons fresh parsley
- 1 tablespoon honey
- 1½ cups filtered water

Method:

1. Add all the ingredients in a high-power blender and pulse until smooth.
2. Pour the smoothie into two glasses and serve immediately.

Nutritional Information per Serving:

- Calories 119
- Total Fat 0.6 g
- Saturated Fat 0.2 g
- Cholesterol 0 mg
- Sodium 42 mg
- Total Carbs 29.5 g
- Fiber 3.4 g
- Sugar 18.6 g
- Protein 3.1 g

Greens & Avocado Smoothie

Preparation Time: 10 minutes

Servings: 2

Ingredients:

- 1 small avocado, peeled, pitted and chopped
- ½ of green bell pepper, seeded and chopped
- 1 cup fresh baby spinach, chopped
- 1 cup fresh arugula, chopped
- 1 (1-inch) fresh ginger piece, peeled and chopped
- ¾ cups fresh parsley
- Pinch of cayenne pepper
- Pinch of salt
- 1 cup fresh coconut water
- ½ cup ice cubes

Method:

1. Add all the ingredients in a high-power blender and pulse until smooth.
2. Pour the smoothie into two glasses and serve immediately.

Nutritional Information per Serving:

- Calories 141
- Total Fat 11.5 g
- Saturated Fat 2.4 g
- Cholesterol 0 mg
- Sodium 127 mg
- Total Carbs 9.8 g
- Fiber 5.5 g
- Sugar 2.3 g
- Protein 2.8 g

Chapter 4: Breakfast Recipes

Blueberry & Ricotta Toast

Preparation Time: 10 minutes
Servings: 2

Ingredients:

- 2 crusty whole-grain bread slices
- ½ cup part-skim ricotta cheese
- 4 tablespoons fresh blueberries
- 2 teaspoons almonds, sliced
- 2 teaspoons honey

Method:

1. Arrange the bread slices onto serving plates.
2. Top each slice with ricotta, followed by blueberries and almonds.
3. Drizzle with honey and serve.

Nutritional Information per Serving:

- Calories 153
- Total Fat 6.3 g
- Saturated Fat 3.2 g
- Cholesterol 19 mg
- Sodium 139 mg
- Total Carbs 16.6 g
- Fiber 0.9 g
- Sugar 8.2 g
- Protein 8.3 g

Berries & Beet Smoothie Bowl

Preparation Time: 10 minutes
Serving: 1

Ingredients:

For Smoothie Bowl:

- 1 cup beets, peeled and chopped
- 1 cup fresh strawberries
- ½ cup fresh cranberries
- 1 scoop vanilla protein powder
- 6 ounces water
- 4 ice cubes

For Topping:

- 2 tablespoons walnuts, chopped
- 1 tablespoon dried cranberries
- 1 tablespoon hemp seeds

Method:

1. For smoothie bowl: add all the ingredients in a high-power blender and pulse until smooth.
2. Pour the smoothie into a serving bowl and top with topping ingredients.
3. Serve immediately.

Nutritional Information per Serving:

- Calories 214
- Total Fat 2.2 g
- Saturated Fat 0.5 g
- Cholesterol 41 mg
- Sodium 164 mg
- Total Carbs 35.4 g
- Fiber 8.3 g
- Sugar 23.5 g
- Protein 12.8 g

Berry Yogurt Bowl

Preparation Time: 10 minutes
Serving: 1

Ingredients:

- ¾ cup fat-free plain Greek yogurt
- ½ cup fresh blueberries
- ½ cup fresh strawberries, hulled and sliced
- 1 tablespoon walnuts, chopped
- 1 teaspoon honey

Method:

1. In a large bowl, place all ingredients except for honey and gently, stir to combine.
2. Drizzle with honey and serve immediately.

Nutritional Information per Serving:

- Calories 265
- Total Fat 7.3 g
- Saturated Fat 2.1 g
- Cholesterol 11 mg
- Sodium 130 mg
- Total Carbs 35.5 g
- Fiber 3.7 g
- Sugar 29.5 g
- Protein 13.4 g

Oatmeal & Yogurt Bowl

Preparation Time: 10 minutes
Cooking Time: 10 minutes
Servings: 2

Ingredients:

- 2 cups water
- 1 cup gluten-free old fashioned oats
- 2 tablespoons tahini
- 1 tablespoon honey
- 1 tablespoon fresh lemon juice
- ¼ teaspoon ground allspice
- 1 (7-ounce) container plain Greek yogurt
- ¼ teaspoon ground cinnamon
- 4 tablespoons fresh blueberries
- 2 tablespoons pistachios, chopped

Method:

1. In a pan, add the water over medium heat and bring to a boil.
2. Stir in the oats and cook about 5 minutes, stirring occasionally.
3. Meanwhile, for sauce: in a small blender, add the tahini, honey, lemon juice and allspice and pulse until smooth.
4. Remove the pan of oats from the heat and stir in half of the yogurt and cinnamon.
5. Divide the oatmeal into serving bowls evenly.
6. Top each bowl with the remaining yogurt, followed by the blueberries and pistachios.
7. Drizzle with the tahini sauce and serve.

Nutritional Information per Serving:

- Calories 375
- Total Fat 14.2 g
- Saturated Fat 2.9 g
- Cholesterol 6 mg

- Sodium 109 mg
- Total Carbs 50 g
- Fiber 6.5 g
- Sugar 18.9 g
- Protein 14.2 g

Overnight Oatmeal

Preparation Time: 10 minutes
Serving: 1

Ingredients:

For Oatmeal:

- ½ cup unsweetened almond milk
- 1 tablespoon maple syrup
- ¾ cup gluten-free old-fashioned oats

For Topping:

- ¼ cup plain Greek yogurt
- ¼ cup fresh strawberries, hulled and sliced
- 3 tablespoons almonds, sliced

Method:

1. In a small bowl, mix the milk and maple syrup.
2. Place the oats into a 1-pint Mason jar and top with almond milk mixture.
3. Cover the jar and refrigerate overnight.
4. In the morning, top the oatmeal with the yogurt, strawberry and almond slices.
5. Serve immediately.

Nutritional Information per Serving:

- Calories 455
- Total Fat 166 g
- Saturated Fat 2.2 g
- Cholesterol 4 mg
- Sodium 135 mg
- Total Carbs 65.8 g
- Fiber 9.5 g
- Sugar 20.2 g
- Protein 15.5 g

Quinoa Porridge

Preparation Time: 10 minutes
Cooking Time: 15 minutes
Servings: 4

Ingredients:

- 1 cup uncooked red quinoa
- 2 cups filtered water
- ½ teaspoon vanilla extract
- ½ cup unsweetened almond milk
- ¼ teaspoon fresh lemon peel, grated finely
- 10-12 drops liquid stevia
- 1 teaspoon ground cinnamon
- ½ teaspoons ground ginger
- ½ teaspoon ground nutmeg
- Pinch of ground cloves
- 1 cup fresh strawberries, hulled and sliced
- ½ cup walnuts, chopped

Method:

1. In a pan, mix together quinoa, water and vanilla extract over low heat and cook for about 15 minutes, stirring occasionally.
2. Add the coconut milk, lemon peel, stevia and spices stir to combine.
3. Immediately, remove from the heat and set aside, covered for about 5 minutes.
4. With a fork, fluff the quinoa.
5. Serve with the topping of strawberries and walnuts.

Nutritional Information per Serving:

- Calories 275
- Total Fat 12.5 g
- Saturated Fat 0.9 g
- Cholesterol 0 mg
- Sodium 26 mg

- Total Carbs 32.8 g
- Fiber 5.3 g
- Sugar 2.1 g
- Protein 10.2 g

Kale & Tomato Scramble

Preparation Time: 10 minutes
Cooking Time: 8 minutes
Servings: 2

Ingredients:

- 1 tablespoon olive oil
- 1 cup fresh baby kale
- 1/3 cup tomato, chopped
- 3 organic eggs, beaten
- 2 tablespoons feta cheese, cubed
- Salt and ground black pepper, as required

Method:

1. In a large frying pan, heat olive oil over medium heat and sauté the kale and tomatoes for about 4 minutes.
2. Add the eggs and cook for about 1 minute, stirring continuously.
3. Stir in the feta and cook for about 2 minutes or until set.
4. Stir in the salt and black pepper and remove from the heat.
5. Serve immediately.

Nutritional Information per Serving:

- Calories 201
- Total Fat 15.6 g
- Saturated Fat 4.5 g
- Cholesterol 254 mg
- Sodium 291 mg
- Total Carbs 5.6 g
- Fiber 0.9 g
- Sugar 1.7 g
- Protein 10.9 g

Eggs with Spinach

Preparation Time: 15 minutes
Cooking Time: 22 minutes
Servings: 2

Ingredients:

- 6 cups fresh baby spinach
- 2-3 tablespoons water
- 4 organic eggs
- Salt and ground black pepper, as required
- 2-3 tablespoons feta cheese, crumbled

Method:

1. Preheat your oven to 400°F.
2. Lightly, grease 2 small baking dishes.
3. In a large frying pan, add spinach and water over medium heat and cook for about 3-4 minutes.
4. Remove from the heat and drain the excess water completely.
5. Divide the spinach into prepared baking dishes evenly.
6. Carefully, crack 2 eggs in each baking dish over spinach.
7. Sprinkle with salt and black pepper and top with feta cheese evenly.
8. Arrange the baking dishes onto a large cookie sheet.
9. Bake for approximately 15-18 minutes.
10. Serve warm.

Nutritional Information per Serving:

- Calories 171
- Total Fat 11.1 g
- Saturated Fat 4.2g
- Cholesterol 336 mg
- Sodium 377 mg
- Total Carbs 4.3 g
- Fiber 2 g
- Sugar 1.4 g
- Protein 15 g

Oatmeal Pancakes

Preparation Time: 15 minutes
Cooking Time: 54 minutes
Servings: 6

Ingredients:

- 1½ cups gluten-free rolled oats
- 2 organic eggs
- 1 ripe banana, peeled
- ¼ cup maple syrup plus extra for drizzling
- 2 tablespoons olive oil
- 1 teaspoon vanilla extract
- 2 teaspoons baking powder
- 2 tablespoons filtered water

Method:

1. Add all the ingredients in a high-power blender and pulse until smooth.
2. Transfer the oatmeal mixture into a bowl.
3. Heat a greased nonstick skillet over medium heat.
4. Place about 1/3 cup of the mixture and with a spatula, spread in an even circle.
5. Cook for about 4-5 minutes.
6. Flip and cook for about 3-4 minutes.
7. Repeat with the remaining mixture.
8. Serve warm with the drizzling of extra maple syrup.

Nutritional Information per Serving:

- Calories 206
- Total Fat 8 g
- Saturated Fat 1.1 g
- Cholesterol 55 mg
- Sodium 23 mg
- Total Carbs 30.3 g
- Fiber 3.1 g
- Sugar 10.4 g
- Protein 5.6 g

Banana & Blueberry Muffins

Preparation Time: 15 minutes
Cooking Time: 22 minutes
Servings: 8

Ingredients:

- ¾ cup oat flour
- ½ cup buckwheat flour
- ½ cup coconut flour
- 1 teaspoon baking powder
- 1 teaspoon baking soda
- 1 teaspoon ground cinnamon
- ¼ teaspoon ground nutmeg
- ¼ teaspoon salt
- 4 ripe bananas, peeled
- ½ cup almond milk
- 1/3 cup coconut oil
- ¼ cup coconut palm sugar
- 1 teaspoon pure vanilla extract
- 2 organic eggs
- 1 cup fresh blueberries
- ¾ cup walnuts, chopped

Method:

1. Preheat your oven to 350°F.
2. Line 16 cups of 2 muffin tins.
3. In a bowl, sift together flours, baking powder, baking soda, spices and salt and mix well.
4. In a separate bowl, place bananas and with a fork, mash well.
5. Add the almond milk, coconut oil, coconut sugar and vanilla extract and beat until well combined.
6. Add eggs, one at a time and beat until well combined.
7. Add the flour mixture and mix until just combined.

8. Gently, fold in the blueberries and walnuts.
9. Transfer the mixture into prepared muffin cups evenly.
10. Bake for approximately 22 minutes or until a wooden skewer inserted in the center comes out clean.
11. Remove the muffin tin from oven and place onto a wire rack to cool for about 10 minutes.
12. Carefully invert the muffins onto the wire rack to cool completely before serving.

Nutritional Information per Serving:

- Calories 346
- Total Fat 19.1 g
- Saturated Fat 9.4 g
- Cholesterol 41 mg
- Sodium 275 mg
- Total Carbs 40.3 g
- Fiber 7.6 g
- Sugar 14 g
- Protein 8.1 g

Chapter 5: Salad Recipes

Berries & Pineapple Salad

Preparation Time: 15 minutes
Servings: 10

Ingredients:

For Salad:

- 1 pineapple, peeled and chopped
- 2 pounds fresh strawberries, hulled and sliced
- 12 ounces fresh blackberries
- 12 ounces fresh blueberries
- 4 cups fresh baby spinach
- 2 ounces Gorgonzola cheese, crumbled

For Dressing:

- ¼ cup white onion, minced
- 1½ teaspoons fresh ginger, grated
- 5½ tablespoons honey
- 1/3 cup apple cider vinegar
- ¼ cup plain Greek yogurt
- ¼ cup olive oil
- 1 teaspoon Dijon mustard
- 1½ teaspoons poppy seeds
- Salt, as required

Method:

1. For salad: in a large salad bowl, mix together all ingredients.
2. For dressing: in a small bowl, add all ingredients and beat well.
3. Place dressing over fruit mixture and toss to coat well.
4. Serve immediately.

Nutritional Information per Serving:

- Calories 219
- Total Fat 7.7 g
- Saturated Fat 1.9 g
- Cholesterol 6 mg
- Sodium 110 mg
- Total Carbs 38.5 g
- Fiber 6.3 g
- Sugar 28.6 g
- Protein 3.9 g

Watermelon & Cucumber Salad

Preparation Time: 15 minutes
Servings: 8

Ingredients:

For Vinaigrette:

- 2 tablespoons fresh lime juice
- 2 tablespoons honey
- 1 tablespoon olive oil
- Pinch of salt

For Salad:

- 1 (5-pound) watermelon, peeled and cut into cubes
- 3 cups cucumber, cubed
- 4 tablespoons fresh mint leaves, torn
- ½ cup feta cheese, crumbled

Method:

1. For vinaigrette: in a small bowl, add all ingredients and beat well.
2. For salad: in a large salad bowl, mix together watermelon, cucumber and mint.
3. Place the vinaigrette over watermelon mixture and gently, toss to coat.
4. Top with the feta cheese and serve immediately.

Nutritional Information per Serving:

- Calories 148
- Total Fat 4.2 g
- Saturated Fat 1.9 g
- Cholesterol 8 mg
- Sodium 130 mg
- Total Carbs 27.7 g
- Fiber 1.5 g
- Sugar 22.8 g
- Protein 3.4 g

Mango, Avocado & Greens Salad

Preparation Time: 20 minutes
Cooking Time: 3 minutes
Servings: 8

Ingredients:

For Dressing:

- 3 tablespoon plus 2 teaspoons olive oil, divided
- 1 cup fresh raspberries
- 1 (¼-inch) piece fresh ginger, chopped
- 2 teaspoons raw honey
- 2 tablespoons fresh lemon juice
- Salt and ground black pepper, as required

For Salad:

- 3 large mangoes, peeled, pitted and cubed
- 1 large avocado, peeled, pitted and sliced
- 12 radishes, trimmed and sliced thinly
- 6 cups fresh baby spinach
- 2 cups watercress leaves
- 3 scallions, sliced thinly
- 3 tablespoons fresh cilantro, chopped
- 2 tablespoons fresh mint leaves, chopped
- 2 tablespoons fresh parsley, chopped
- ½ cup sunflower seeds, shelled and toasted

Method:

1. For dressing: in a small frying pan, heat 2 teaspoons of oil over medium heat and cook the raspberries for about 3 minutes, stirring occasionally.
2. Remove the frying pan from heat and set aside to cool slightly.
3. In a blender, add cooked raspberries and remaining oil and all ingredients and pulse till smooth.
4. For salad: in a large salad bowl, add all ingredients except sunflower seeds and mix.

5. Place raspberry dressing over salad and toss to coat well.
6. Serve immediately with the garnishing of sunflower seeds.

Nutritional Information per Serving:

- Calories 222
- Total Fat 13.3 g
- Saturated Fat 2.2 g
- Cholesterol 0 mg
- Sodium 51 mg
- Total Carbs 26.7 g
- Fiber 6 g
- Sugar 20 g
- Protein 3.5 g

Greens Salad

Preparation Time: 15 minutes
Servings: 2

Ingredients:

- 4 cups mixed baby greens (spinach, kale, arugula etc.)
- 1 cup cucumber, julienned
- ¼ cup carrot, peeled and julienned
- 1 tablespoon fresh lemon juice
- 1 tablespoon olive oil
- Salt and ground black pepper, as required
- ¼ cup hummus

Method:

1. In a large salad bowl, add greens, cucumber, carrot, lemon juice, oil, salt and black pepper and toss to coat well.
2. Drizzle with hummus and serve.

Nutritional Information per Serving:

- Calories 150
- Total Fat 10.1 g
- Saturated Fat 1.5 g
- Cholesterol 0 mg
- Sodium 306 mg
- Total Carbs 12.3 g
- Fiber 4 g
- Sugar 1.7 g
- Protein 4.5 g

Chickpeas & Couscous Salad

Preparation Time: 20 minutes
Cooking Time: 5 minutes
Servings: 6

Ingredients:

- 1½ cups vegetable broth
- 1 teaspoon ground cumin
- 1½ cups uncooked couscous
- ½ cup raisins
- 1 (16-ounce) can chickpeas, rinsed and drained
- 3 medium tomato, chopped
- 2 scallions, sliced
- 2 tablespoons fresh parsley, chopped
- 2 tablespoons fresh mint leaves, chopped
- 2 teaspoon fresh orange zest, grated
- 3-4 tablespoons fresh orange juice
- 1 tablespoon olive oil

Method:

1. In a small saucepan, add broth and cumin and bring to a boil.
2. Stir in couscous and immediately remove from the heat.
3. Cover the saucepan and set aside for about 5 minutes.
4. Uncover the pan and with a fork, fluff the couscous.
5. Transfer the couscous into a bowl.
6. Add remaining ingredients and gently stir to combine.
7. Serve immediately.

Nutritional Information per Serving:

- Calories 305
- Total Fat 3.8 g
- Saturated Fat 0.5 g
- Cholesterol 0 mg

- Sodium 262 mg
- Total Carbs 58.2 g
- Fiber 6.2 g
- Sugar 10.4 g
- Protein 10.1 g

Pasta & Tomato Salad

Preparation Time: 20 minutes
Cooking Time: 10 minutes
Servings: 4

Ingredients:

For Salad

- ½ cup uncooked whole-wheat orzo pasta
- 3 plum tomatoes, chopped
- 1 cup black olives, pitted and sliced
- 6 cups fresh spinach, chopped roughly
- 3 scallions, chopped
- ½ cup feta cheese, crumbled
- 1 tablespoon capers, drained

For Dressing

- 1/3 cup olive oil
- 4 teaspoons fresh lemon juice
- 1 tablespoon fresh parsley, minced
- 2 teaspoons fresh lemon zest, grated
- Salt and ground black pepper, as required

Method:

1. For salad: in a large pan of the salted boiling water, cook the orzo for about 8-10 minutes or until according to package's instructions.
2. Drain the orzo and rinse under cold running water.
3. In a large salad bowl, add pasta and remaining ingredients and mix.
4. For dressing: in a small bowl, add all ingredients and beat until well combined.
5. Place the dressing over salad and toss to coat well.
6. Refrigerate to chill completely before serving.

Nutritional Information per Serving:

- Calories 340

- Total Fat 25.1 g
- Saturated Fat 5.8 g
- Cholesterol 17 mg
- Sodium 648 mg
- Total Carbs 25.2 g
- Fiber 4.4 g
- Sugar 4.1 g
- Protein 7.9 g

Nutty Chicken Salad

Preparation Time: 20 minutes
Servings: 6

Ingredients:

For Dressing:

- 2-3 tablespoons plain Greek yogurt
- 3 tablespoons Dijon mustard
- 2 tablespoons sunflower seeds
- 1 teaspoon kelp powder
- ½ teaspoon ground turmeric
- ¼ teaspoon garlic powder
- ¼ teaspoon onion powder
- Salt and ground black pepper, as required

For Salad:

- 4 (6-ounce) cooked chicken breasts, shredded
- 2-3 celery stalks, chopped
- 2 tablespoons fresh parsley, chopped
- ¼ cup dried cherries
- ¼ cup almonds, chopped
- 6 cups fresh baby kale

Method:

1. For dressing: in a bowl, add all ingredients and beat until well combined.
2. For salad: in a large serving bowl, add all the ingredients and mix.
3. Place dressing over the salad and gently, toss to coat.
4. Serve immediately.

Nutritional Information per Serving:

- Calories 340
- Total Fat 25.1 g
- Saturated Fat 5.8 g

- Cholesterol 17 mg
- Sodium 648 mg
- Total Carbs 25.2 g
- Fiber 4.4 g
- Sugar 4.1 g
- Protein 7.9 g

Chicken & Veggies Salad

Preparation Time: 20 minutes
Servings: 6

Ingredients:

For Salad:

- 3 cups cooked chicken breast, cubed
- 2 cups tomatoes, chopped
- 1 cup Kalamata olives, pitted
- ½ cup red onion, chopped finely
- ½ cup feta cheese, crumbled

For Dressing:

- ¼ cup olive oil
- 2 tablespoons fresh lemon juice
- 1 tablespoon fresh cilantro, minced
- Salt and ground black pepper, as required

Method:

1. For salad: in a large salad bowl, mix together all ingredients.
2. For dressing: in a small bowl, add all ingredients and beat well.
3. Place dressing over salad and toss to coat well.
4. Refrigerate to chill completely before serving.

Nutritional Information per Serving:

- Calories 252
- Total Fat 15.7 g
- Saturated Fat 4.1 g
- Cholesterol 65 mg
- Sodium 410 mg
- Total Carbs 5.3 g
- Fiber 1.7 g
- Sugar 2.6 g
- Protein 22.9 g

Salmon & Beans Salad

Preparation Time: 15 minutes
Servings: 2

Ingredients:

- 8 ounces cooked wild salmon
- ½ cup canned white beans, drained and rinsed
- ½ cup cooked green beans, cut in 2-inch pieces
- ½ cup cherry tomatoes, halved
- 2 large organic hard-boiled eggs, sliced
- 1 tablespoon olive oil
- 2 teaspoons lemon juice
- 4 cups fresh baby spinach

Method:

1. In a large salad bowl, add all ingredients except for spinach and toss to coat well.
2. Serve salad over spinach leaves.

Nutritional Information per Serving:

- Calories 415
- Total Fat 22.3 g
- Saturated Fat 4.3 g
- Cholesterol 256 mg
- Sodium 202 mg
- Total Carbs 16.9 g
- Fiber 7.8 g
- Sugar 2.8 g
- Protein 36.8 g

Tuna Salad

Preparation Time: 20 minutes
Servings: 6

Ingredients:

For Vinaigrette:

- 3 tablespoons fresh lime juice
- 1/3 cup olive oil
- 2½ teaspoons Dijon mustard
- 1 teaspoon fresh lime zest, grated
- Salt and ground black pepper, as required

For Salad:

- 3 (5-ounce) cans tuna in olive oil
- 1 red onion, chopped
- 2 cucumbers, sliced
- 1 large tomato, sliced
- ½ cup Kalamata olives, pitted
- 8 cups fresh spinach leaves, torn
- ¼ cup fresh basil leaves

Method:

1. For vinaigrette: in a bowl, add all ingredients and beat until well combined.
2. For salad: in a large serving bowl, add all the ingredients and mix.
3. Place vinaigrette over the salad and gently, toss to coat.
4. Refrigerate, covered for about 30-40 minutes before serving.

Nutritional Information per Serving:

- Calories 280
- Total Fat 18.6 g
- Saturated Fat 3 g
- Cholesterol 22 mg
- Sodium 220 mg

- Total Carbs 9 g
- Fiber 2.6 g
- Sugar 3.5 g
- Protein 21.3 g

Chapter 6: Lunch Recipes

Pita Sandwiches

Preparation Time: 20 minutes
Cooking Time: 8 minutes
Servings: 4

Ingredients:

For Chicken Marinade:

- 2 tablespoons fresh lemon juice
- 3 teaspoons olive oil
- 1 tablespoon fresh oregano, chopped
- 1½ teaspoons garlic, minced
- 1 teaspoon lemon zest
- Salt ground black pepper, as required
- 1-pound chicken tenders

For Yogurt Sauce:

- 1 English cucumber, seeded and grated,
- Salt, as required
- ¾ cup nonfat plain Greek yogurt
- 2 teaspoons olive oil
- 2 teaspoons fresh dill, chopped
- 2 teaspoons fresh mint, chopped
- ½ teaspoons garlic, minced
- Ground black pepper, as required

For Sandwiches:

- 2 (6½-inch) whole-wheat pita breads, halved
- 1 cup fresh spinach, torn
- 1 cup plum tomatoes, chopped
- ½ of English cucumber, halved and sliced

- ½ cup red onion, sliced

Method:

1. For marinade: in a large ceramic bowl, add all ingredients except for chicken and mix well.
2. Add chicken tenders and toss to coat.
3. Cover the bowl and refrigerate to marinate for about 2 hours.
4. Meanwhile, for yogurt sauce: in a strainer, place the cucumber and sprinkle with ¼ teaspoon of salt.
5. Set aside to drain for 15 minutes.
6. With your hands, squeeze the cucumber to release the liquid.
7. Transfer the cucumber into a medium bowl.
8. Add the remaining sauce ingredients and stir to combine.
9. Refrigerate the sauce until ready to serve.
10. Preheat the grill to medium-high heat. Lightly, grease the grill grate.
11. Remove the chicken tenders from the bowl and shake off excess marinade.
12. Place the chicken tenders onto the grill and cook for about 3-4 minutes per side.
13. Spread some of sauce inside each pita half.
14. Fill each pita half with chicken, spinach, tomato, cumber and onion.
15. Serve with the topping of any remaining sauce.

Nutritional Information per Serving:

- Calories 427
- Total Fat 16.1 g
- Saturated Fat 3.9 g
- Cholesterol 104 mg
- Sodium 357 mg
- Total Carbs 30.7 g
- Fiber 4.6 g
- Sugar 8.1 g
- Protein 40.6 g

Veggie Tortillas

Preparation Time: 20 minutes
Cooking Time: 5 minutes
Servings: 2

Ingredients:

- ½ teaspoon olive oil
- ½ of small zucchini, sliced thinly
- ½ of medium red bell pepper, seeded and sliced thinly
- 1 red onion, sliced thinly
- 2 whole-grain tortillas
- ¼ cup hummus
- ½ cup fresh baby spinach
- 2 tablespoons feta cheese, crumbled
- 1 teaspoon dried oregano
- 1 tablespoon black olives, pitted and sliced

Method:

1. Heat the olive oil in a small skillet over medium-low heat and sauté the zucchini, bell pepper and onion for about 5 minutes.
2. Meanwhile, in another nonstick skillet, heat the tortillas until warmed.
3. Place the hummus onto the center of each wrap evenly and top with spinach, followed by the sautéed vegetables, feta, oregano and olives.
4. Carefully, fold the edges of each tortilla over the filling to roll up.
5. Cut each roll in half cross-wise and serve.

Nutritional Information per Serving:

- Calories 282
- Total Fat 10.4 g
- Saturated Fat 3.6 g
- Cholesterol 8 mg
- Sodium 592 mg
- Total Carbs 39.2 g

- Fiber 8.4 g
- Sugar 6.8 g
- Protein 10.4 g

Chickpeas Wraps

Preparation Time: 20 minutes
Cooking Time: 25 minutes
Servings: 2

Ingredients:

For Wraps:

- 1 (15-ounce) can chickpeas, drained, rinsed and pat dried
- 1 tablespoon olive oil
- ½ teaspoon garlic powder
- ¼ teaspoon smoked paprika
- ¼ teaspoon ground cumin
- 4 large lettuce leaves
- 1 avocado, peeled, pitted and chopped
- 1 cup cherry tomatoes, halved

For Sauce:

- ¼ cup water
- ½ cup cashews, soaked for at least 2 hours and drained
- 1 teaspoon capers
- 3 tablespoons fresh lemon juice
- 1 tablespoon tahini
- 2 garlic cloves, peeled
- 2 tablespoons unsweetened almond milk
- ½ teaspoon Dijon mustard
- Salt, as required

Method:

1. Preheat your oven to 400 °F.
2. Line a baking sheet with parchment paper.
3. In a bowl, add the chickpeas, oil, spices and salt and toss to coat well.
4. Arrange the chickpeas onto the prepared baking sheet in an even layer.
5. Bake for approximately 20-25 minutes or until crispy.

6. Meanwhile, for sauce: in a high-speed blender, add all ingredients and pulse until smooth.
7. Transfer the sauce into a bowl and set aside.
8. Arrange the lettuce leaves onto serving plates.
9. Divide the chickpeas, avocado and tomatoes over each leaf evenly.
10. Drizzle with sauce and serve immediately.

Nutritional Information per Serving:

- Calories 631
- Total Fat 41.3 g
- Saturated Fat 7.6 g
- Cholesterol 0 mg
- Sodium 428 mg
- Total Carbs 52.9 g
- Fiber 13.1 g
- Sugar 6.1 g
- Protein 18.5 g

Meatballs & Quinoa Bowl

Preparation Time: 20 minutes
Cooking Time: 15 minutes
Servings: 4

Ingredients:

For Meatballs:

- 1 pound 93%-lean ground turkey
- 1 cup frozen chopped spinach, thawed and squeezed
- ½ cup feta cheese, crumbled
- ½ teaspoon garlic powder
- ½ teaspoon dried oregano
- Salt ground black pepper, as required
- 2 tablespoons olive oil

For Quinoa Bowl:

- 2 cups cooked and cooled quinoa
- 2 cups cucumber, sliced
- 2 cups cherry tomatoes
- ½ cup fresh parsley, chopped
- 3 tablespoons fresh mint, chopped
- 2 tablespoons fresh lemon juice
- 1 tablespoon olive oil

Method:

1. For meatballs: place all ingredients except for oil in a bowl and mix until well combined.
2. Make 12 equal-sized meatballs form the mixture.
3. Heat the olive oil in a large nonstick skillet over medium heat and cook the meatballs for about 10-15 minutes or until done completely, flipping occasionally.
4. With a slotted spoon, transfer the meatballs onto a plate and set aside to cool.
5. For quinoa bowl, in a large bowl, mix together all ingredients.
6. Divide quinoa mixture onto 4 serving plates and top each with meatballs.

7. Serve immediately.

Nutritional Information per Serving:

- Calories 556
- Total Fat 23.3 g
- Saturated Fat 6 g
- Cholesterol 123 mg
- Sodium 381 mg
- Total Carbs 52.2 g
- Fiber 7.7 g
- Sugar 6.2 g
- Protein 38.1 g

Turkey Burgers with Green Sauce

Preparation Time: 15 minutes
Cooking Time: 8 minutes
Servings: 4

Ingredients:

For Burgers:

- 1 (2-inch) piece fresh ginger, grated
- 1 pound lean ground turkey
- 1 medium onion, grated
- 2 garlic cloves, minced
- 1 bunch fresh mint leaves, chopped finely
- 2 teaspoons ground coriander
- 2 teaspoons ground cumin
- ½ teaspoon ground allspice
- ½ teaspoon ground cinnamon
- Salt and ground black pepper, as required
- 1 tablespoon olive oil

For Serving:

- 1 large avocado, peeled, pitted and chopped
- 6 cups fresh baby greens
- 2 tablespoons olive oil
- 1 tablespoon fresh lemon juice
- Salt and ground black pepper, as required

Method:

1. Preheat the broiler of oven.
2. Lightly, grease a broiler pan.
3. For burgers in a large bowl, squeeze the juice of ginger.
4. Add remaining ingredients and mix till well combined.
5. Make equal sized burgers from the mixture.

6. Arrange the burgers onto the prepared broiler pan and broil for about 5 minutes per side.
7. Meanwhile, for serving: in a bowl, add all ingredients and toss to coat well.
8. Divide avocado mixture and burgers onto serving plates and serve.

Nutritional Information per Serving:

- Calories 381
- Total Fat 28.8 g
- Saturated Fat 6.2 g
- Cholesterol 81 mg
- Sodium 138 mg
- Total Carbs 9.8 g
- Fiber 5 g
- Sugar 2.1 g
- Protein 24.5 g

Lentil Falafel Bowl

Preparation Time: 20 minutes
Cooking Time: 20 minutes
Servings: 4

Ingredients:

For Falafel:

- 4 tablespoons fresh parsley
- 1 small red onion, chopped roughly
- 2 garlic cloves, peeled
- 1 cup red lentils, soaked overnight
- 2 tablespoons chickpea flour
- 2 tablespoons fresh lemon juice
- 2 tablespoons olive oil
- ½ teaspoon ground cumin
- Salt and ground black pepper, as required

For Dressing:

- ¼ cup tahini
- 2 garlic cloves, minced
- 2 tablespoons fresh lemon juice
- 1 tablespoon white miso
- ¼ cup filtered water

For Salad:

- 1 cup green olives, pitted
- 3 large tomatoes, sliced
- 5 cups fresh baby spinach

Method:

1. Preheat your oven to 400 °F.
2. Line a baking sheet with parchment paper.

3. For falafel: in a food processor, add the parsley, onion and garlic and pulse until finely chopped.
4. Now, place the remaining ingredients and pulse until just combined.
5. Make small sized patties from the mixture.
6. Arrange the patties onto the prepared baking sheet in a single layer.
7. Bake for approximately 18-20 minutes or until patties become golden brown.
8. For dressing: in a bowl, add all the ingredients and beat until well combined.
9. Divide salad ingredients and falafel patties into serving bowls evenly.
10. Drizzle with dressing and serve immediately.

Nutritional Information per Serving:

- Calories 437
- Total Fat 20.5 g
- Saturated Fat 3 g
- Cholesterol 0 mg
- Sodium 557 mg
- Total Carbs 48.5 g
- Fiber 21.5 g
- Sugar 6.9 g
- Protein 19.8 g

Chicken & Veggie Skewers

Preparation Time: 20 minutes
Cooking Time: 10 minutes
Servings: 6

Ingredients:

- 5 tablespoons fresh lemon juice
- ¼ cup olive oil
- 2 garlic cloves, minced
- 1 teaspoon ground cumin
- 1 teaspoon dried oregano
- ½ teaspoon dried thyme
- Salt and ground black pepper, as required
- 2 pounds skinless, boneless chicken breast, cut into 1½-inch pieces
- 2 large green bell peppers, seeded and cut into 1-inch pieces
- 12 fresh mushrooms
- 12 cherry tomatoes
- 1 large onion, quartered and separated into pieces

Method:

1. In a large ceramic bowl, add lemon juice, oil, garlic, cumin, oregano, herbs salt and black pepper and beat until well combined.
2. Add the chicken pieces and toss to coat well.
3. With a plastic wrap, cover the bowl and refrigerate to marinate for at least 2 hours.
4. Preheat an outdoor grill to medium-high heat. Lightly, grease the grill grate.
5. Remove the chicken pieces from the bowl and shake off excess marinade.
6. Thread the chicken pieces and vegetables onto the pre-soaked wooden skewers.
7. Place the skewers onto the grill and cook for about 10 minutes, turning frequently.
8. Serve hot.

Nutritional Information per Serving:

- Calories 304
- Total Fat 14.3 g

- Saturated Fat 3.4 g
- Cholesterol 88 mg
- Sodium 90 mg
- Total Carbs 8.7 g
- Fiber 2 g
- Sugar 4.8 g
- Protein 36.1 g

Nutty Quinoa

Preparation Time: 10 minutes
Cooking Time: 25 minutes
Servings: 4

Ingredients:

- 2 tablespoons olive oil
- 1 teaspoon curry powder
- 1 teaspoon ground turmeric
- ½ teaspoon ground cumin
- 1 cup uncooked quinoa, rinsed and drained
- 2 cups chicken broth
- ¾ cup almonds, toasted
- ½ cup raisins
- ¾ cup fresh parsley, chopped

Method:

1. In a medium saucepan, heat oil on medium-low heat and sauté the curry powder, turmeric and cumin for about 1-2 minutes.
2. Add the quinoa and sauté for about 2-3 minutes.
3. Add broth and stir to combine.
4. Adjust the heat to low and simmer, covered for about 20 minutes.
5. Remove the saucepan from heat and set aside, covered for about 5 minutes.
6. In the pan of quinoa mixture, add almonds and raisins and toss to coat.
7. Drizzle with lemon juice and serve.

Nutritional Information per Serving:

- Calories 402
- Total Fat 19.5 g
- Saturated Fat 2.2 g
- Cholesterol 0 mg
- Sodium 393 mg
- Total Carbs 47.4 g

- Fiber 6.6 g
- Sugar 12 g
- Protein 13.2 g

Chapter 7: Dinner Recipes

Lentils & Spinach Soup

Preparation Time: 15 minutes
Cooking Time: 1¼ hours
Servings: 6

Ingredients:

- 2 tablespoons olive oil
- 2 carrots, peeled and chopped
- 2 celery stalks, chopped
- 2 sweet onions, chopped
- 3 garlic cloves, minced
- 1½ cups brown lentils, rinsed
- 2 cups tomatoes, chopped finely
- ¼ teaspoon dried basil, crushed
- ¼ teaspoon dried oregano, crushed
- ¼ teaspoon dried thyme, crushed
- 1 teaspoon ground cumin
- ½ teaspoon ground coriander
- 6 cups vegetable broth
- 3 cups fresh spinach, chopped
- Salt and ground black pepper, as required
- 2 tablespoons fresh lemon juice

Method:

1. In a large soup pan, heat the oil over medium heat and sauté carrot, celery and onion for about 4-5 minutes.
2. Add the garlic, sauté for about 1 minute.
3. Add the lentils and sauté for about 2-3 minutes.
4. Stir in the tomatoes, herbs, spices and broth and bring to a boil.
5. Adjust the heat to low and simmer, partially covered for about 45-60 minutes.
6. Stir in the spinach, salt and black pepper and cook for about 3-4 minutes.

7. Stir in the lemon juice and serve hot.

Nutritional Information per Serving:

- Calories 291
- Total Fat 6.9 g
- Saturated Fat 1.2 g
- Cholesterol 0 mg
- Sodium 830 mg
- Total Carbs 39 g
- Fiber 7.2 g
- Sugar 6.1 g
- Protein 19 g

Chicken & Chickpeas Stew

Preparation Time: 20 minutes
Cooking Time: 1 hour 5 minutes
Servings: 12

Ingredients:

- 5 pounds skinless, boneless chicken thighs, trimmed
- Salt and ground black pepper, as required
- ¼ cup olive oil
- 3 large yellow onions, sliced thinly
- 8 garlic cloves, crushed
- 2 fresh bay leaves
- 1 tablespoon ground turmeric
- 2 teaspoon ground coriander
- 2 teaspoons ground cumin
- 2 (3-inch) cinnamon sticks
- 4 teaspoons fresh lemon zest, grated finely
- ½ cup fresh lemon juice, divided
- 4 cups low-sodium chicken broth
- 2 cups small green olives, pitted
- 2 cups canned chickpeas, rinsed and drained
- ½ cup fresh cilantro, chopped

Method:

1. Sprinkle the chicken thighs with salt and black pepper evenly.
2. In a large soup pan, heat the oil over medium-high heat.
3. Add the chicken thighs in 2 batches and cook for about 3 minutes per side.
4. With a slotted spoon, transfer the chicken thighs into a bowl and set aside.
5. In the same pan, add the onion over medium heat and sauté for about 5-6 minutes.
6. Add the garlic, bay leaves and spices and sauté for about 1 minute.
7. Add the lemon zest, 1/3 cup of the lemon juice and broth and bring to a boil.
8. Adjust the heat to medium-low and simmer, covered for about 30 minutes.
9. Add the cooked chicken, olives and chickpeas and stir to combine.

10. Adjust the heat to medium-high and cook for about 6-8 minutes, stirring occasionally.
11. Stir in remaining lemon juice, salt and black pepper and remove from heat.
12. Serve hot with the garnishing of cilantro.

Nutritional Information per Serving:

- Calories 449
- Total Fat 15.6 g
- Saturated Fat 3.8 g
- Cholesterol 110 mg
- Sodium 311 mg
- Total Carbs 27 g
- Fiber 7.6 g
- Sugar 5.5 g
- Protein 5.2 g

Chickpeas & Veggie Curry

Preparation Time: 20 minutes
Cooking Time: 30 minutes
Servings: 6

Ingredients:

- 6 tablespoons olive oil, divided
- 2 carrots, peeled and chopped
- 1 sweet potato, peeled and cubed
- 1 medium eggplant, cubed
- 1 red bell pepper, seeded and chopped
- 1 green bell pepper, seeded and chopped
- 1 onion, chopped
- 3 garlic cloves, minced
- 1 tablespoon curry powder
- 1 teaspoon ground turmeric
- 1 teaspoon ground cinnamon
- Salt and ground black pepper, as required
- 1 (15-ounce) can chickpeas, drained and rinsed
- 1 zucchini, sliced
- 1 cup fresh orange juice
- ¼ cup blanched almonds
- 2 tablespoons raisins
- 10 ounces fresh spinach

Method:

1. In a large Dutch oven, heat 3 tablespoons of oil over medium heat and sauté the carrots, sweet potato, eggplant, bell peppers and onion for about 5 minutes.
2. Meanwhile, in another medium pan, heat remaining oil over medium heat and sauté the garlic, curry powder, cinnamon, turmeric, salt and black pepper for about 3 minutes.
3. Transfer the garlic mixture into the pan of the vegetables and stir to combine.

4. Stir in the chickpeas, zucchini, orange juice, almonds and raisins and simmer, covered for about 20 minutes.
5. Stir in the spinach and cook, uncovered for about 5 minutes.
6. Serve hot.

Nutritional Information per Serving:

- Calories 322
- Total Fat 17.7 g
- Saturated Fat 2.2 g
- Cholesterol 0 mg
- Sodium 259 mg
- Total Carbs 38 g
- Fiber 10 g
- Sugar 15 g
- Protein 8.1 g

Braised Chicken

Preparation Time: 15 minutes
Cooking Time: 1 hour
Servings: 6

Ingredients:

- 6 (8-ounce) bone-in chicken thighs
- Salt and ground black pepper, as required
- 2 tablespoons olive oil
- ½ of onion, sliced
- 4 cups chicken broth
- ½ teaspoon ground turmeric
- 8 sprigs fresh dill
- 2 tablespoons fresh lemon juice
- 2 tablespoons arrowroot starch
- 1 tablespoon filtered water
- ½ tablespoon fresh dill, chopped

Method:

1. Sprinkle the chicken thighs with salt and black pepper.
2. In a large nonstick skillet, heat the olive oil over high heat.
3. Place the chicken thighs in skillet, skin side down and cook for about 3-4 minutes.
4. With a slotted spoon, transfer the thighs onto a plate.
5. In the same skillet, add onion over medium heat and sauté for about 4-5 minutes.
6. Return the thighs in skillet, skin side up with broth, turmeric, salt and black pepper.
7. Place the dill sprigs and over thighs and bring to a boil.
8. Adjust the heat to medium-low and simmer, covered for about 40-45 minutes, coating the thighs with cooking liquid.
9. Meanwhile, in a small bowl, mix together arrowroot starch and water.
10. Discard the thyme sprigs and transfer the thighs into a bowl.
11. Add the lemon juice in sauce and stir to combine.
12. Slowly, add the arrowroot starch mixture, stirring continuously.

13. Cook for about 3-4 minutes or until desired thickness, stirring occasionally.
14. Serve hot with the topping of chopped dill.

Nutritional Information per Serving:

- Calories 514
- Total Fat 22.5 g
- Saturated Fat 5.6 g
- Cholesterol 202 mg
- Sodium 735 mg
- Total Carbs 4.6 g
- Fiber 0.5 g
- Sugar 1 g
- Protein 69.2 g

Roasted Chicken

Preparation Time: 15 minutes
Cooking Time: 1 hour 40 minutes
Servings: 5

Ingredients:

- ¼ cup olive oil
- 3 garlic cloves, minced
- 2 teaspoons lemon zest, grated finely
- 2 teaspoons dried oregano, crushed
- 1 teaspoon paprika
- 1 teaspoon ground cumin
- Salt and ground black pepper, as required
- 1 (3-pound) frying chicken, neck and giblets removed

Method:

1. In a large bowl, add all ingredients except the chicken and mix well.
2. Add the chicken and coat with the mixture generously.
3. Refrigerate to marinate overnight, turning occasionally.
4. Preheat your oven to 425 °F.
5. Remove the chicken from the bowl and arrange in a roasting pan.
6. Coat the chicken with the remaining marinade.
7. With a kitchen string, tie the legs and tuck the wings back under the body.
8. Roast for about 10 minutes.
9. Now, reduce the temperature of oven to 350 °F and roast for about 1½ hours.
10. Remove the roasting pan from oven and place the chicken onto a cutting board for about 10 minutes before carving.
11. Cut into desired sized pieces and serve.

Nutritional Information per Serving:

- Calories 505
- Total Fat 18.6 g
- Saturated Fat 3.8 g

- Cholesterol 210 mg
- Sodium 204 mg
- Total Carbs 1.6 g
- Fiber 0.6 g
- Sugar 0.1 g
- Protein 79.2 g

Salmon with Capers

Preparation Time: 10 minutes
Cooking Time: 8 minutes
Servings: 4

Ingredients:

- 2 tablespoons olive oil
- 4 (6-ounce) salmon fillets
- 2 tablespoons capers
- Salt and ground black pepper, as required
- 4 lemon wedges

Method:

1. In a large nonstick skillet, heat oil over high heat and cook the salmon fillets for about 3 minutes.
2. Sprinkle the salmon fillets with capers, salt and black pepper.
3. Flip the salmon fillets and cook for about 5 minutes or until browned.
4. Serve with the garnishing of lemon wedges.

Nutritional Information per Serving:

- Calories 286
- Total Fat 17.5 g
- Saturated Fat 2.5 g
- Cholesterol 75 mg
- Sodium 241 mg
- Total Carbs 0.4 g
- Fiber 0.2 g
- Sugar 0.1 g
- Protein 33.1 g

Salmon with Avocado Cream

Preparation Time: 15 minutes
Cooking Time: 8 minutes
Servings: 4

Ingredients:

For Avocado Cream:

- 2 avocados, peeled, pitted and chopped
- 1 cup plain Greek yogurt
- 2 garlic cloves, chopped
- 3-4 tablespoons fresh lime juice
- Salt and ground black pepper, as required

For Salmon:

- 2 teaspoons ground cumin
- 2 teaspoons garlic powder
- Salt and ground black pepper, as required
- 4 (6-ounce) skinless salmon fillets
- 2 tablespoons olive oil

Method:

1. For avocado cream: in a food processor, add all the ingredients and pulse until smooth.
2. In a small bowl, mix together the spices, salt and black pepper.
3. Coat the salmon fillets with spice mixture evenly.
4. In a nonstick skillet, heat the olive oil over medium-high heat and cook salmon fillets for about 3 minutes.
5. Flip and cook for about 4-5 minutes or until desired doneness.
6. Transfer the salmon fillets onto serving plates.
7. Top with avocado cream and serve.

Nutritional Information per Serving:

- Calories 685

- Total Fat 49.9 g
- Saturated Fat 9.8 g
- Cholesterol 95 mg
- Sodium 293 mg
- Total Carbs 15 g
- Fiber 7 g
- Sugar 5.2 g
- Protein 46.4 g

Tuna with Olives Sauce

Preparation Time: 15 minutes
Cooking Time: 32 minutes
Servings: 4

Ingredients:

- 6 tablespoons olive oil
- 1 large yellow onion, chopped
- 3 garlic cloves, minced and divided
- 1 cup Roma tomato, chopped
- 8 fresh basil leaves, chopped
- 4 tablespoons fresh parsley, chopped and divided
- 4 (8-ounce) tuna steaks
- Salt and ground black pepper, as required
- 1 cup black olives, pitted and sliced
- 4 teaspoons capers, rinsed

Method:

1. In a large nonstick skillet, heat 3 tablespoons of olive oil over medium heat and sauté the onion for about 3 minutes.
2. Add 2 garlic cloves and sauté for about 2 minutes.
3. Stir in the tomatoes, basil and 2 tablespoons of parsley and cook for about 15 minutes, stirring occasionally.
4. Meanwhile, season the tuna steaks with salt and black pepper evenly.
5. In another large skillet, heat the remaining olive oil over medium heat and sauté the remaining garlic for about 1 minute.
6. Place the tuna steaks in a single layer.
7. Adjust the heat to medium-high and cook for about 2 minutes, stirring occasionally.
8. Place the tomato mixture, olives and capers over tuna steaks and gently stir to combine.
9. Adjust the heat to low and cook for about 5 minutes.
10. Garnish with remaining parsley and serve.

Nutritional Information per Serving:

- Calories 486
- Total Fat 26.8 g
- Saturated Fat 3.5 g
- Cholesterol 99 mg
- Sodium 509 mg
- Total Carbs 8.5 g
- Fiber 2.7 g
- Sugar 2.8 g
- Protein 5.4 g

Chicken with Spinach & Pasta

Preparation Time: 15 minutes
Cooking Time: 10 minutes
Servings: 4

Ingredients:

- 8 ounces whole-wheat penne pasta
- 2 tablespoons olive oil
- 1 pound boneless, skinless chicken breasts, trimmed and cut into bite-size pieces
- Salt and ground black pepper, as required
- 4 garlic cloves, minced
- ½ cup chicken broth
- 3 tablespoons fresh lemon juice
- 2 teaspoons lemon zest, grated
- 10 cups fresh spinach, chopped

Method:

1. In a large pan of lightly salted boiling water, add the pasta and cook for about 8-10 minutes or according to package's directions.
2. Drain the pasta well.
3. Meanwhile, heat oil in a large high-sided skillet over medium-high heat and cook the chicken with salt and black pepper for about 5-7 minutes, stirring occasionally.
4. Add garlic and cook for about 1 minute, stirring continuously.
5. Stir in broth, lemon juice and zest; bring to a simmer.
6. Stir in the spinach and cooked pasta and remove from the heat.
7. Immediately, cover the skillet and set aside for about 3-4 minutes before serving.

Nutritional Information per Serving:

- Calories 494
- Total Fat 17 g
- Saturated Fat 3.5 g
- Cholesterol 101 mg
- Sodium 304 mg

- Total Carbs 38.1 g
- Fiber 7.8 g
- Sugar 0.7 g
- Protein 44.8 g

Lentil & Quinoa Casserole

Preparation Time: 20 minutes
Cooking Time: 50 minutes
Servings: 6

Ingredients:

- 2 tablespoons olive oil
- 1 large yellow onion, chopped
- 3 garlic cloves, minced
- 10 ounces fresh baby spinach
- 2½ cups cooked quinoa
- 1½ cups cooked brown lentils
- 2 cups cherry tomatoes, halved
- 2 medium organic eggs
- ½ cup plain, non-fat Greek yogurt
- 6 ounces feta cheese, crumbled
- ½ cup fresh dill, chopped
- Salt and ground black pepper, as required

Method:

1. Preheat your oven to 375 °F.
2. Grease a 9x13-inch casserole dish.
3. In a large skillet, heat olive oil over medium heat and sauté the onion and garlic for about 3-5 minutes.
4. Stir in the spinach and cook, covered for about 2-2½ minutes.
5. Uncover and cook for about 2-2½ minutes.
6. With a slotted spoon, transfer the spinach mixture onto a paper towels-lined plate to drain.
7. In a large bowl, add the quinoa, lentils, spinach mixture and tomatoes and mix.
8. In another large bowl, add the yogurt, eggs, feta, dill, salt and black pepper and mix until well combined.
9. Add the quinoa mixture and mix until well combined.
10. Place the mixture into the prepared casserole dish evenly.

11. Bake for approximately 35-40 minutes or until top becomes golden brown.
12. Remove the casserole dish from oven and set aside to cool for about 10 minutes before serving.

Nutritional Information per Serving:

- Calories 573
- Total Fat 17 g
- Saturated Fat 5.6 g
- Cholesterol 81 mg
- Sodium 448 mg
- Total Carbs 76 g
- Fiber 14.5 g
- Sugar 8.1 g
- Protein 3.8 g

Chapter 8: Snack Recipes

Roasted Chickpeas

Preparation Time: 10 minutes
Cooking Time: 45 minutes
Servings: 8

Ingredients:

- 4 cups cooked chickpeas
- 2 garlic cloves, minced
- ½ teaspoon dried oregano, crushed
- ½ teaspoon smoked paprika
- ¼ teaspoon ground cumin
- Salt, as required
- 1 tablespoon olive oil

Method:

1. Preheat your oven to 400 °F.
2. Grease a large baking sheet.
3. Place chickpeas onto the prepared baking sheet and spread in a single layer.
4. Roast for about 30 minutes, stirring after every 10 minutes.
5. Meanwhile, in a small bowl, mix together garlic, thyme and spices.
6. Remove the baking sheet from oven.
7. Place the garlic mixture and oil over the chickpeas and toss to coat well.
8. Roast for approximately 10-15 minutes more.
9. Now, turn the oven off but leave the baking sheet inside for about 10 minutes before serving.

Nutritional Information per Serving:

- Calories 147
- Total Fat 2.8 g
- Saturated Fat 0.3 g
- Cholesterol 0 mg

- Sodium 50 mg
- Total Carbs 21.4 g
- Fiber 5.1 g
- Sugar 0 g
- Protein 7.1 g

Roasted Nuts

Preparation Time: 10 minutes
Cooking Time: 12 minutes
Servings: 16

Ingredients:

- 1½ cups whole almonds
- 1½ cups pistachios
- 1½ cups walnut halves
- 1½ cup cashews
- 1/3 cup olive oil
- 2 tablespoons fresh rosemary, chopped
- 2 tablespoons fresh thyme, chopped
- 2 tablespoons fresh oregano, chopped
- 1 tablespoon smoked paprika
- 1 teaspoon ground cumin
- 2 teaspoons garlic powder
- Salt, as required

Method:

1. Preheat your oven to 350 °F.
2. Line a large baking sheet with a parchment paper.
3. In a bowl, place all ingredients and toss to coat well.
4. Transfer the nut mixture onto the prepared baking sheet and spread in a single layer.
5. Roast for about 10-12 minutes, flipping after every 5 minutes.
6. Remove from the oven and set the baking sheet aside to cool completely before serving.

Nutritional Information per Serving:

- Calories 271
- Total Fat 24.4 g
- Saturated Fat 2.9 g

- Cholesterol 0 mg
- Sodium 45 mg
- Total Carbs 10.2 g
- Fiber 3.6 g
- Sugar 1.7 g
- Protein 8.1 g

Chocolate Oatmeal Cookies

Preparation Time: 15 minutes
Cooking Time: 13 minutes
Servings: 7

Ingredients:

- 1 cup gluten-free quick oats
- ¾ cup whole-wheat flour
- 1½ teaspoons baking powder
- 1½ teaspoons ground cinnamon
- ½ teaspoon salt
- 1 large organic egg
- ½ cup honey
- 2 tablespoons coconut oil, melted and cooled
- 1 teaspoon vanilla extract
- ½ cup dark chocolate chips

Method:

1. Preheat your oven to 325 °F.
2. Line a large baking sheet with parchment paper.
3. Place oats, flour, baking powder, cinnamon and salt and mix well.
4. In a separate bowl, place egg, honey, coconut oil and vanilla extract and beat until well combined.
5. Add flour mixture and mix until just combined.
6. Gently, fold in the chocolate chips.
7. Refrigerate the dough for about 30 minutes.
8. Preheat your oven to 325 °F.
9. Line a large cookie sheet with parchment paper.
10. Place 14 cookies onto prepared cookie sheet about 2-inch apart.
11. Bake for approximately 12-13 minutes or until golden brown.
12. Remove from oven and place the cookie sheet onto a wire rack to cool for about 5 minutes.
13. Now, invert the cookies onto the wire rack to cool before serving.

Nutritional Information per Serving:

- Calories 261
- Total Fat 7.9 g
- Saturated Fat 5.2 g
- Cholesterol 27 mg
- Sodium 179 mg
- Total Carbs 45.2 g
- Fiber 2.1 g
- Sugar 24.9 g
- Protein 4.9 g

Tuna Croquettes

Preparation Time: 20 minutes
Cooking Time: 29 minutes
Servings: 8

Ingredients:

- ¼ cup plus 1 tablespoon olive oil, divided
- ½ of large onion, chopped
- 1 (1-inch) piece fresh ginger, minced
- 3 garlic cloves, minced
- 1 Serrano pepper, seeded and minced
- ½ teaspoon ground coriander
- ¼ teaspoon ground turmeric
- ¼ teaspoon red chili powder
- Salt and ground black pepper, as required
- 2 (5-ounce) cans tuna
- 1 cup cooked sweet potato, peeled and mashed
- 1 organic egg
- ¼ cup tapioca flour
- ¼ cup almond flour

Method:

1. In a frying pan, heat 1 tablespoon of olive oil over medium heat and sauté the onion, ginger, garlic and Serrano pepper for about 5-7 minutes.
2. Stir in spices and sauté for about 1 minute more.
3. Transfer the onion mixture into a bowl.
4. Add tuna and sweet potato and mix until well combined.
5. Make equal sized oblong shaped patties from the mixture.
6. Arrange the croquettes onto a baking sheet in a single layer and refrigerate for overnight.
7. In a shallow dish, beat the egg.
8. In another shallow dish mix together both flours.

9. In a deep skillet, heat the remaining olive oil over medium heat and shallow fry the croquettes in 2 batches and for about 2-3 minutes per side.

Nutritional Information per Serving:

- Calories 249
- Total Fat 13.9 g
- Saturated Fat 2.1 g
- Cholesterol 31 mg
- Sodium 57 mg
- Total Carbs 20.4 g
- Fiber 1.5 g
- Sugar 2.1 g
- Protein 11.6 g

Oats & Pistachio Bars

Preparation Time: 15 minutes
Servings: 8

Ingredients:

- 20 dates, pitted
- 1¼ cups pistachios, roasted
- 1 cup gluten-free rolled old fashioned oats
- 2 tablespoons almond butter
- ¼ cup unsweetened applesauce
- 1 teaspoon vanilla extract

Method:

1. In a food processor, add dates and pulse until pureed.
2. Add pistachios and oats and pulse until crumbly mixture is formed.
3. Place the almond butter, applesauce and vanilla extract and pulse until a slightly sticky dough forms.
4. Place the mixture into an 8x8-inch parchment paper-lined baking dish.
5. With the back of a spoon, press down the top surface firmly.
6. Arrange a parchment paper on top of mixture and freeze for at least 1 hour before cutting.
7. With a knife, cut into 8 bars and serve.

Nutritional Information per Serving:

- Calories 175
- Total Fat 7.5 g
- Saturated Fat 0.8 g
- Cholesterol 0 mg
- Sodium 51 mg
- Total Carbs 26.5 g
- Fiber 4.1 g
- Sugar 15.1 g
- Protein 4.5 g

Date & Pistachio Bites

Preparation Time: 15 minutes
Servings: 16

Ingredients:

- 2 cups dates, pitted
- 1 cup raw unsalted pistachios, shelled
- 1 cup golden raisins
- 1 teaspoon ground fennel seeds
- 1/8 teaspoon ground black pepper

Method:

1. In a food processor, add all ingredients and pulse until finely chopped.
2. Make about 32 balls from the mixture and arrange onto 2 parchment paper-lined baking sheets in a single layer.
3. Refrigerate until set completely before serving.

Nutritional Information per Serving:

- Calories 110
- Total Fat 1.9 g
- Saturated Fat 0.2 g
- Cholesterol 0 mg
- Sodium 21 mg
- Total Carbs 24.9 g
- Fiber 2.5 g
- Sugar 19.7 g
- Protein 1.6 g

Dates & Oat Bites

Preparation Time: 15 minutes
Servings: 11

Ingredients:

- 1 cup dates, pitted
- ½ cup gluten-free old-fashioned rolled oats
- ¼ cup chia seeds
- ¼ cup pecans, chopped
- 2 medium carrots, peeled and chopped finely
- 1 teaspoon vanilla extract
- ¾ teaspoon ground cinnamon
- ½ teaspoon ground ginger
- ¼ teaspoon ground turmeric
- ¼ teaspoon salt
- Pinch of ground black pepper

Method:

1. In a food processor, add dates, oats, chia seeds and pecans and pulse until finely chopped.
2. Add remaining ingredients and pulse until a paste begins to form.
3. Make about 32 balls from the mixture and arrange onto 2 parchment paper-lined baking sheets in a single layer.
4. Refrigerate until set completely before serving.

Nutritional Information per Serving:

- Calories 98
- Total Fat 3.5 g
- Saturated Fat 0.3 g
- Cholesterol 0 mg
- Sodium 62 mg
- Total Carbs 17.5 g
- Fiber 3.3 g
- Sugar 11.1 g
- Protein 1.9 g

Chickpeas Hummus

Preparation Time: 10 minutes
Servings: 12

Ingredients:

- 4 cups cooked chickpeas
- ½ cup tahini
- 1 garlic clove, chopped
- 2 tablespoons fresh key lime juice
- Salt, as required
- Water, as required
- 1 tablespoon olive oil
- Pinch of cayenne powder

Method:

1. In a blender, add all ingredients and pulse until smooth.
2. Transfer the hummus into a large bowl and drizzle with oil.
3. Sprinkle with cayenne powder and serve immediately.

Nutritional Information per Serving:

- Calories 137
- Total Fat 7.5 g
- Saturated Fat 0.9 g
- Cholesterol 0 mg
- Sodium 210 mg
- Total Carbs 13.6 g
- Fiber 3.6 g
- Sugar 1.3 g
- Protein 5 g

Beans & Spinach Dip

Preparation Time: 10 minutes
Servings: 8

Ingredients:

- 1 (15-ounce) can cannellini beans, rinsed and drained
- ½ cup fresh spinach
- ½ of large ripe avocado, peeled, pitted and chopped
- 2 garlic cloves, chopped
- 2-3 tablespoons fresh lime juice
- 2 tablespoons fresh cilantro
- 2 tablespoons olive oil
- Salt, as required

Method:

1. In a blender, add all ingredients and pulse until smooth.
2. Transfer the dip into a large bowl and serve.

Nutritional Information per Serving:

- Calories 230
- Total Fat 6 g
- Saturated Fat 1 g
- Cholesterol 0 mg
- Sodium 35 mg
- Total Carbs 33.2 g
- Fiber 14 g
- Sugar 1.3 g
- Protein 12.9 g

Olives & Tomato Salsa

Preparation Time: 15 minutes
Servings: 4

Ingredients:

- 12 ounces cherry tomatoes, quartered
- 2 shallots, chopped finely
- 6 kalamata olives, pitted and chopped
- 1 garlic clove, minced
- ½ cup fresh mint, chopped
- ½ cup fresh parsley, chopped
- 2 teaspoons olive oil
- 2 teaspoons lemon juice
- Salt and ground black pepper, as required

Method:

1. In a large bowl, place all the ingredients and gently toss to coat well.
2. Set aside for about 10-15 minutes before serving.

Nutritional Information per Serving:

- Calories 59
- Total Fat 3.4 g
- Saturated Fat 0.5 g
- Cholesterol 0 mg
- Sodium 110 mg
- Total Carbs 7 g
- Fiber 2.3 g
- Sugar 2.4 g
- Protein 1.7 g

Chapter 9: Dessert Recipes

Stuffed Apples

Preparation Time: 15 minutes
Cooking Time: 35 minutes
Servings: 4

Ingredients:

- 4 large apples, peeled and cored
- 2 teaspoons fresh lemon juice
- 1 cup fresh blueberries
- ½ cup fresh apple juice
- ½ teaspoon ground cinnamon
- ¼ cup almond meal
- ¼ cup coconut flakes

Method:

1. Preheat your oven to 375 °F.
2. Brush the apples with lemon juice evenly and arrange in a baking dish.
3. Stuff each apple with blueberries.
4. Scatter the remaining blueberries around the apples.
5. Drizzle with apple juice and sprinkle each apple with cinnamon evenly.
6. Top with almond meal and coconut flakes evenly.
7. Bake for approximately 30-35 minutes.
8. Serve warm.

Nutritional Information per Serving:

- Calories 204
- Total Fat 5.2 g
- Saturated Fat 1.7 g
- Cholesterol 0 mg
- Sodium 5 mg
- Total Carbs 41.9 g

- Fiber 7.7 g
- Sugar 30.4 g
- Protein 2.4 g

Frozen Strawberry Yogurt

Preparation Time: 15 minutes
Servings: 4

Ingredients:

- 4 cups frozen strawberries
- 1/3 cups plain Greek yogurt
- 2 tablespoons honey
- 1 teaspoon pure vanilla extract
- 1 teaspoon fresh lemon juice
- Pinch of salt
- 1 tablespoon fresh mint leaves

Method:

1. In a food processor, add all ingredients except the mint and pulse until smooth.
2. Serve immediately with the garnishing of mint leaves.

Nutritional Information per Serving:

- Calories 96
- Total Fat 0.7 g
- Saturated Fat 0.2 g
- Cholesterol 0 mg
- Sodium 1 mg
- Total Carbs 21.4 g
- Fiber 3 g
- Sugar 17.3 g
- Protein 2.2 g

Chocolaty Cherry Ice Cream

Preparation Time: 15 minutes
Servings: 2

Ingredients:

- 1 cup raw cashews
- 1 cup frozen cherries
- ¼ cup unsweetened coconut, shredded
- 1 tablespoon raw honey
- ¼ cup dark chocolate, chopped

Method:

1. In a high-speed blender, add cashews and pulse until a flour like texture forms.
2. Add remaining ingredients except chocolate and pulse until smooth.
3. Add chocolate and pulse until just combined.
4. Transfer the ice-cream into airtight container and freeze for about 1-2 hours or until set.

Nutritional Information per Serving:

- Calories 635
- Total Fat 35.7 g
- Saturated Fat 11.4 g
- Cholesterol 5 mg
- Sodium 20 mg
- Total Carbs 69.6 g
- Fiber 6.4 g
- Sugar 50.3 g
- Protein 13.5 g

Avocado Mousse

Preparation Time: 15 minutes
Servings: 4

Ingredients:

- 2 cups bananas, peeled and chopped
- 2 ripe avocados, peeled, pitted and chopped
- 1 teaspoon fresh lime zest, grated finely
- 1 teaspoon fresh lemon zest, grated finely
- ½ cup fresh lime juice
- ½ cup fresh lemon juice
- 1/3 cup honey

Method:

1. In a blender, add all ingredients and pulse until smooth.
2. Transfer the mousse in 4 serving glasses and refrigerate to chill for about 3 hours before serving.

Nutritional Information per Serving:

- Calories 337
- Total Fat 17.1 g
- Saturated Fat 3.8 g
- Cholesterol 0 mg
- Sodium 13 mg
- Total Carbs 48.8 g
- Fiber 7.9 g
- Sugar 33.5 g
- Protein 2.8 g

Chocolate Cake

Preparation Time: 15 minutes
Cooking Time: 29½ minutes
Servings: 8

Ingredients:

- 7 ounces dark chocolate, chopped finely
- ½ cup olive oil
- 1 cup coconut palm sugar
- 5 large organic eggs
- 1 teaspoon vanilla extract
- 4 tablespoons cacao powder
- 1 teaspoon espresso powder
- ¼ teaspoon salt

Method:

1. Preheat your oven to 350 °F.
2. Line the bottom of a lightly greased round 9-inch cake pan with parchment paper.
3. In a microwave-safe bowl, add chocolate and olive oil and microwave on High for about 60-90 seconds, stirring after every 30 seconds.
4. Remove from microwave and stir the mixture until smooth.
5. Set aside to cool for 2-3 minutes.
6. In a large bowl, add chocolate mixture and coconut sugar and beat well.
7. Add the eggs, one at a time and beat until well combined.
8. Add the vanilla and mix well.
9. Add cocoa powder, espresso powder and salt and mix until just combined.
10. Place the mixture into the prepared cake pan evenly.
11. Bake for approximately 25-28 minutes or until a wooden skewer inserted in the center comes out clean.
12. Remove from the oven and place the cake pan onto a wire rack for about 10 minutes.
13. Carefully, remove the cake from the pan and place onto the wire rack to cool completely before serving.

14. Cut into desired-sized slices and serve.

Nutritional Information per Serving:

- Calories 383
- Total Fat 23.6 g
- Saturated Fat 8.2 g
- Cholesterol 122 mg
- Sodium 191 mg
- Total Carbs 40.4 g
- Fiber 1.6 g
- Sugar 31.1 g
- Protein 6.3 g

Conclusion

Now you that the PAMM diet not only offers wide-ranging health benefits but also offers a variety of ingredients, flavors, and aromas. Relatively simple and basic, in essence, this diet is worthy of trying. And this book has given you all the reason to do so, with its range of delicious and flavorsome recipes. Now with the PAMM diet, you can enjoy all the Mediterranean and Asian flavors packed into a single cuisine. Choosing variety will not make you compromise on the quality, as long as you are choosing the right ingredients. Bring the much-needed balance in your diet and try all the PAMM diet recipes shared in this book. Soon, you will witness all the promising health benefits of this super-healthy diet.

CPSIA information can be obtained
at www.ICGtesting.com
Printed in the USA
LVHW062250231020
669603LV00012B/164